YOUR KNOWLEDGE HAS VALUE

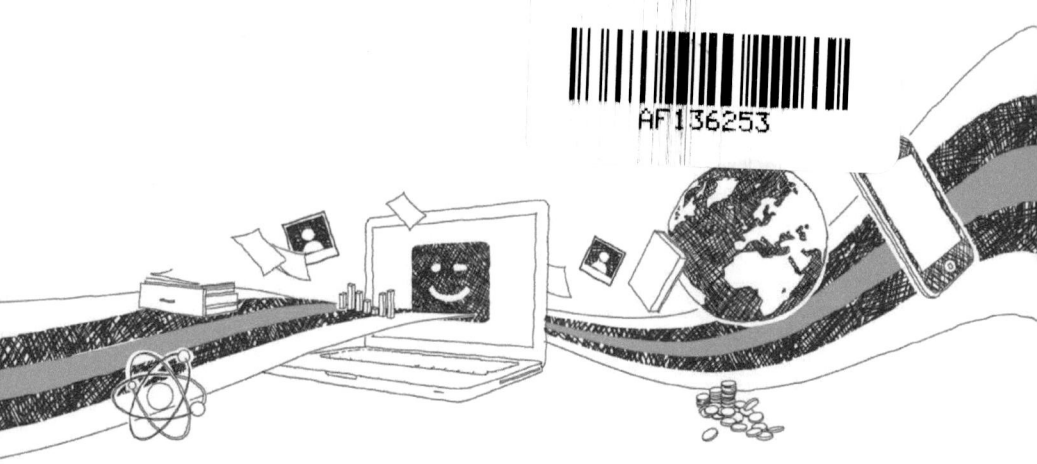

- We will publish your bachelor's and master's thesis, essays and papers

- Your own eBook and book - sold worldwide in all relevant shops

- Earn money with each sale

Upload your text at www.GRIN.com and publish for free

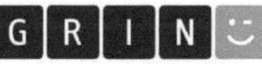

Bibliographic information published by the German National Library:

The German National Library lists this publication in the National Bibliography; detailed bibliographic data are available on the Internet at http://dnb.dnb.de .

Imprint:

Copyright © 2020 GRIN Verlag
Print and binding: Books on Demand GmbH, Norderstedt Germany
ISBN: 9783346245199

This book at GRIN:

https://www.grin.com/document/585133

Dina Were, Joel Ogutu

Suicidal behaviour among Kenyan youth. Risk factors and prevalence in secondary schools

A short research

GRIN Verlag

GRIN - Your knowledge has value

Since its foundation in 1998, GRIN has specialized in publishing academic texts by students, college teachers and other academics as e-book and printed book. The website www.grin.com is an ideal platform for presenting term papers, final papers, scientific essays, dissertations and specialist books.

Visit us on the internet:

http://www.grin.com/

http://www.facebook.com/grincom

http://www.twitter.com/grin_com

RISK FACTORS AND PREVALENCE OF SUICIDAL BEHAVIOUR AMONG KENYAN YOUTH IN SECONDARY SCHOOLS

Joel Peter Ogutu
Masinde Muliro University of Science and Technology
Department of Educational Psychology

Dinah Shisia Were
Kaimosi Friends University College
(A Constitute College of Masinde Muliro University of Science and Technology)

Abstract

The occurrence of reported suicide cases amongst young people in Kenya is alarming and yet many cases go unreported in most cultures in Kenya due social stigma associated with suicide. It is worth noting that suicide in Kenya has become more rampant among the youth than adults and that the majority of reported suicide cases happen amongst youth in high schools, colleges and universities. The aim of this study was to establish risk factors associated with increased cases of suicide in a sample representative among Kenyan young people.

Methods: *Participants were drawn from university and high school students. Among other instrument, they completed Beck Scale for Suicide Ideation (BSS).*

Results: *The dysfunctional family, church, academic pressure media, depression, and relationship problems were risk factors that laid the foundation for suicidal behavior among youths. Suicidal behaviours included thoughts, plans and attempts. The society is becoming more individualistic and hence most people suffer in silence.*

Conclusion: *Suicidal behaviour among youth in secondary schools poses a significant challenge to mental health practices in learning institutions of Kenya. The findings are relevant for promotion of mental health programmes in public learning institutions and professional training facilities in relevant sectors, especially in counseling, health and social workers.*

Key words: Behaviour, prevalence, risk factors, suicidal behaviour, youth, mental health

Table of Contents

1. Introduction

Suicide is a major health problem, and the global suicide mortality rate amounts to 1.4% of all deaths worldwide. Most suicides are related to psychiatric disease, with depression, substance use disorders and psychosis being the most relevant risk factors (Heu, Bogren, Wong, Brådvik, et al 2018). However, anxiety, personality, eating, and trauma related disorders, as well as organic mental disorders, also contribute.

Suicide is a mental health problem that offers a permanent solution to a temporary problem in a flashflood of negative emotions. Suicide is the result of a convergence of risk factors including but not limited to genetic, psychological, social and cultural risk factors, sometimes combined with experiences of trauma and loss, with depression as the most common mental disorder in people who die by suicide (WHO, 2019). According to the World Health Organization (WHO) during 2019 world suicide prevention day reported that about 800,000 people die from suicide each year (that is one person every 40 seconds), majority of them being youth aged 15-29 year. For every 1 suicide 25 people make a suicide attempt. That has made suicide one of the leading causes of death. It was further revealed by WHO that each year, the proportion of suicides accounts for more deaths than war and homicide combined. Increased suicide cases among young people indicate failure to address growing gaps in mental health services for young people globally.

Also, 90 per cent of suicides among youth are related to mental disorders, including depression, and substance abuse. Suicide among youth is a silent mental illness since it remains undiagnosed and undermanaged. World Health Organization (2019) has cited insufficient resources, ineffective coordination, lack of policy guideline and independent and systematic evaluation as challenges to curbing suicides. As UNICEF (2012) asserts, Adolescents experience intense physical, psychological, emotional and economic changes as they make the transition from childhood to adulthood.

Several studies have also indicated that suicidal ideation among youth may be increasing (Spirito & Esposito-Smythers, 2006; Cash & Bridge, 2009). A recent nationally representative survey of school aged adolescents (approximately 14-18 years) in the United States showed that in the 12 months prior to the survey, 15% had reported suicidal ideation while 7% reported having made a suicide attempt (Eaton *et al.*,2008).

While there may be unique risk factors for suicidal behaviors and death among youth in sub-Saharan Africa, previous research shows that living on the streets (Iemmi, 2016), substance use (Page, 2011), adverse childhood experiences (King, 2008), and HIV/AIDS, sexually transmitted (Ng, 2015) and sexually transmitted infections (STIs) (Swahn, 2012) are important risk factors for suicidality among youth

In addition, in a research conducted among sub-Saharan African adolescents, Palmier (2011) showed that East African countries are not immune from the endemic tragedy of suicide. According to the study, Zambia had the highest prevalence of suicidal ideation (31.9%), followed by Kenya (27.9%), Botswana (23.1%), Uganda (19.6%) and Tanzania (11.2%) among youth who eventually committed suicide. The prevalence of suicidal ideation in Botswana, Kenya, Uganda and Zambia was higher (19.6%-31.9%) than in the U.S. (16.9%) and Europe as seen in prior studies (Swahn et al, 2012). In a similar research conducted in Nigeria among 1,429 adolescent students by Omigbodun, Dogra, Esan, and Adedokun (2008), over 20% of the students reported suicidal ideation while 12% reported that they had attempted suicide in the previous year. The research also indicated that adolescents in urban areas, especially from polygamous or disrupted families, had higher rates of suicidal behavior. Many developed countries have initiated national suicide prevention programme while African countries are still lagging behind

In Kenyan a day rarely goes without media reporting on suicide case of youth due to being shamed and ridiculed by peers and teachers like the case of a primary school girl who committed suicide after allegedly ridiculed by her teacher for soiling her clothes with menses. The girl's death prompted protests from parents, and the wider Kenyan population about how the teacher chose to handle the situation. Official numbers on suicide in Kenya may be difficult to get due to apparent under-reporting or misreporting of such deaths, in part because there are penalties in Kenyan law for attempting suicide, as well as higher levels of stigmatization. Yet, it is clear that deaths from suicide deal a devastating blow to families, friends, and communities.

2. Literature review

2.1 Mental disorders and suicide

Foster et al, (2018) carried out a study on prevalence of disorders among suicidal youth in Northern Ireland. The aim of this part of the Northern Ireland Suicide Study was to investigate the prevalence of DSM - III - R axis I (clinical syndrome) and axis II (personality) disorders among suicides (14 years and older) in Northern Ireland during a one-year period. The method used was a psychological autopsy study based on a variety of documentary sources and interviews with bereaved informants and health care professionals. The results were that Ninety per cent of suicides (106/118) had a current axis I and/or an axis II mental disorder. At least one current axis I disorder was diagnosed in 86% of suicides (102/118), and at least one axis II disorder was diagnosed in 44% (52/118). Suicides under 30 years (92% male) were less likely to have a current axis I disorder (68%; 26/38) than those 30 years and older (95%; 76/80). Psychiatric comorbidity was present in 55% of suicides (65/118). The time between the last contact with a health care professional and death was greater among suicides under 30 years and male suicides. They concluded that notwithstanding the etiological complexity of suicide, the prevention, recognition and treatment of mental disorder will continue to play key roles in suicide prevention.

Researchers have indicated that suicidal behaviors among adolescents are clearly associated with mental disorders. Miller et al. (2007) noted that over 90% of adolescents completing suicide had a mental illness at the time of their death. Further, according to Miller et al (2007) younger adolescents completing suicide tend to have higher rates of mental illness. Similarly, another study revealed a relationship between suicide behaviors and mental disorder. Also, 90 per cent of suicides among youth are related to mental disorders, including depression, and substance abuse. Suicide among youth is a silent mental illness since it remains undiagnosed and undermanaged (World Health Organization, 2019).

Adolescents with at least one diagnosed mental disorder were four times more likely to attempt suicide than those with no disorder. On the other hand, youths with three or more disorders were eight times more likely to attempt suicide or develop suicidal ideation than those with no psychiatric disorders (Khasakhala et al, 2011). Therefore, this research sought to establish the severity of suicide behaviors among adolescents at Federal Neuropsychiatric

Hospital, Kappa-Lagos, Nigeria. This study site is one of the referral Federal psychiatric hospitals in Nigeria and the only one in Lagos State.

Tanney, (1992) explores the value of psychiatric disorders as a predictive variable for suicide by addressing recent evidence concerning the relationship between psychiatric disorders and suicide / a general discussion of the definition and classification of psychiatric disorders and of suicidal behaviors is provided at the outset / then recent studies investigating the link or association between psychiatric disorders and suicide are summarized, with special attention to the relationships between specific disorders and suicide / various explanations addressing the nature of the association or relationship are proposed / finally, some broad conclusions about the value of psychiatric information in the assessment and prediction of suicide are offered.

Lönnqvist et al, (1995) in the research phase of the National Suicide Prevention Project, all suicides (n= 1397) in Finland between March 1987 and April 1988 were examined retrospectively using the psychological autopsy method. Careful retrospective diagnostic evaluation of the victims according to DSM-III-R criteria was done by weighing and integrating all available information. A series of studies addressing the mental disorders among suicide victims, the treatment received before death and the life events is now reviewed. Among a random sample of suicide victims from the nationwide suicide population, at least one psychiatric diagnosis was made for 93% of the victims. The most prevalent disorders were depressive syndromes (66%) and alcohol dependence/abuse (43%). The prevalence of major depression was higher among women than among men. Major depression as the principal diagnosis was more common among the elderly suicides. Among adolescent victims, depressive syndromes were also the most prevalent disorders. Adjustment disorders were common (25%) among male adolescent suicides. The majority of suicide victims of all ages suffered from comorbid mental disorders.

2.2   Family issues and suicide

A study indicated that lack of parent-child bond could lead to confusion, conflict and frustration in the growing child. This, according to them, serves as an antecedent for an adolescent to develop psychopathology and suicidal behavior (Khasakhala et al, 2013). In addition, Linehan (2015) noted that suicidal behavior is a response to unbearable emotional

6

suffering. In Uganda, suicidal ideation was associated with problem drinking and a range of adverse childhood experiences such as physical abuse, orphan hood, homelessness, and rape (Culbreth et al, 2018).

It was observed that depression is also known to be the most common disorder among people who die by suicide. In a review a few years ago, the risk factors in this disorder were family history of psychiatric disorders, male gender, suicide attempts, more severe depression, hopelessness and co morbidity. This was based on 19 studies (28 papers), which is a surprisingly low number considering the high suicide risk in the disorder (Hawton et al, 2013).

2.3   Cultural issues and suicide

Magaya etal (2005), in a study among a sample of Zimbabwean adolescents, found out that cultural factors bear a significant influence on adolescents' choice of coping approaches, as adolescents are often encouraged to adopt non-confrontational and avoidant behaviors that are focused on the promotion of a harmonious and interdependent social environment. This may result into bottling up anger, unvented rage and suicidal ideation. Though this study was done in Zimbabwe, the Kenyan communities, especially in the rural areas bring up their children in a similar way. It would therefore be important to find out whether teachers know that how students have been socialized to deal with stressing events is related to suicidal behavior.

According to a review, most studies on ethnicity/immigrant status and suicide attempts showed higher rates among immigrants as compared to the native population, Forte et al, (2018), though the reverse was found in a few cases. Risk factors were found to be: language barriers, worrying about family back home and separation from family, often leading to hopelessness, depression, and anxiety. Furthermore, the lack of information on the health care system, loss of status, loss of social network, as well as acculturation when an individual acquires attitudes, etc. from a different country were identified as potential triggers to suicide. Unlike American culture as a whole, "Asian cultures condone and accept the practice of suicide as legitimate in the context of familial shame, interpersonal conflict, and for altruistic reasons," observed Aruna, LCSW, research assistant professor, University of Illinois at Chicago. "When informed of a death by suicide, Asians are more likely to say it was understandable."

7

More than one million individuals worldwide die by suicide annually. Although suicide exists in every country, religious group, and age group, suicidal behavior is "differently determined and has different meanings in different cultures." Yet, despite the clear role of culture in suicidal behavior, it is often neglected by clinicians (Molock et al, 2020). Certain risk factors depression, anxiety, and mental illness are common in all cultural groups. In contrast, among blacks suicide is taboo. Suicide is seen as a sin, and the spiritual and cultural norms are often regarded as protective. But those same norms may prevent people from getting help because even suicidal ideation is regarded as taboo. Like, Asian cultures tend to be other-focused and community based (Molock, 2020).

2.4 Health and suicide

Prior study from USA inform that adolescents who struggle with suicidal behavior often exhibit unhealthy thought patterns due to mental health issues such as depression, that lead to thoughts of hopelessness, helplessness, and worthlessness (SAMHSA, 2012). In china, factors identified with suicidal ideation include poor family structure and parental relationship

Handley et al (2018) noted that as part of the Australian Rural Mental Health Study, the relationship between depression and suicidal behaviour be investigated. They found out that of 1051 participants, 364 reported life-time depression. Of these, 48% reported life-time suicidal ideation and 16% reported a life-time suicide attempt. The severity of depression was a significant correlate of suicidality in both men and women, but suicide attempts were significantly more common among females with a younger age of depression onset, and a higher number of psychiatric comorbidities. No additional factors were found for males, which agrees with the study on ACE above (Cleare et al (2018).Prediction may be more difficult in men, and they more often die by their own hand (Crona et al, 2017).

2.5 Psychology and suicide

As UNICEF (2012) asserts, Adolescents experience intense physical, psychological, emotional and economic changes as they make the transition from childhood to adulthood. The youth of (13-19 years) are mostly in Secondary Schools where they spend most of their time yet this is the peak age of suicide attempts. They deal with major psychological tasks that

8

accompany this phase under reduced dependence on their parents and separated from the family and forming an adult identity.

Macharia (2013) in a study on suicidal behavior risk factors of secondary schools adolescents in in Nyandarua, Kenya, found that parent-child communication, dysfunctional families, irresponsible parenting, absence of parents and parents pressure on adolescents to perform academically were risk factors that fuelled suicide ideation among adolescents. The adolescents also learned suicidal behaviour from family members Mental health experts, assert that increased rate of attempted suicide cases among young people in Kenya is due to limited capacity to think, act and process emotion in a rational manner especially when exposed to unbearable pressure, stress, drugs and alcohol. Among the Kenyan youth, Suicidal behaviour is a common problem among youths identified with psychiatric or substance abuse disorder (Lincoln et al (2013).

According to Schlebusch et al (2009), young people employ suicidal behavior as more desperate cry for help and a first-line, crisis-management technique. This, he explains, is consistent with international research which indicates that a substantial proportion of people who commit or attempt suicide indicate a need for help. Lack of interpersonal problem solving skills too increases the adolescents' risk to suicide. He adds that a knowledgeable teacher would not dismiss suicidal behavior as indiscipline; rather seek to understand the cause for that suicidal behavior.

Cleare et al (2018) state that adverse childhood experiences (ACE) have been implicated in a range of negative health outcomes in adulthood, including mental disorders and suicide death. One paper explores the relationship between ACE and hospital-treated self-harm in Glasgow. First-time and repeat self-harm were compared, including mental health, psychosocial measures, and attachment style. However, only ACE along with female gender and depressive symptoms differentiated between first-time and repeat self-harm. Participants with 4+ ACE were significantly more likely to repeat. There were no differentiating factors in the male group. The findings stress the importance of ACE as a risk factor for suicidal behaviour, but more research is needed for the male group (Cleare et al (2018).

2.6   Academics and suicide

Symptoms that may be readily observed in the school setting include an inability to concentrate, to think rationally, or make even minor decisions; other observable symptoms include difficulty getting necessary things done, self-harm behavior, withdrawing from normal relationships or isolating oneself, and increased absenteeism in school (Klein et al., 2013). Such problems may be reflected in students' classroom behavior, homework habits, and academic performance (Hubert, 2006).

According to police reports, majority of suicide cases are secondary school students and primary school pupils who kill themselves in depression-fueled impulses and academic performance related circumstances. From Bungoma county in Kenya, a form one student from a Girls High School committed suicide using a piece of a bed sheet in her dormitory after allegedly being paraded before other students and shamed over claims of altering her Geography marks. He said that the deceased left behind a suicide note stating that she did not cheat in Geography and would rather die than being shamed before fellow students.

Police report from Kakamega county in Kenya indicate that between 2017 and 2018 at least 50 people committed suicide in the county. For instance, a 12 year, Class Seven pupil at a Kakamega Primary School, hanged himself inside their house. A 17 years old Form Three student at Girls High School, strangled herself using a necktie. According to a suicide note addressed to her sister, she decided to kill herself after being suspended from school. In Busia County Kenya, a form one student at Secondary School was found hanging from a rope that was tied to the roof at her lover's house. A young boy threatened to commit suicide when his family failed to raise school fees to enable him join High School after scoring 345 marks in Kenya Certificate of Primary School (KCPE) examination.

Other causes are linked to disappointment with academic performances, bullying from their peers, relationship break-up or loss and a sense of isolation. Another case was where a student committed suicide when a phone confiscated by her teacher was thrown in a pit latrine.

2.7   Cyber bulling and suicide

A systematic review on self-harm, suicidal behaviours, and cyber bullying in Children and Young People authored by Ann et al (1996) revealed that cyber bulling contributes to self harm and suicide. Following concerns about bullying via electronic communication in children and young people and its possible contribution to self-harm, a review of the evidence for associations between cyber bullying involvement and self-harm or suicidal behaviors (such as suicidal ideation, suicide plans, and suicide attempts) in children and young people was done. Aboujaoude et al (2015), in their review on cyber bullying as an old problem gone viral observed some personality disorders as a result of cyber bulling. They stated that cyber bullying should also be considered as a cause for new onset psychological symptoms, somatic symptoms of unclear etiology or a drop in academic performance. The aim of the study was to systematically review the current evidence examining the association between cyber bullying involvement as victim or perpetrator and self-harm and suicidal behaviors in children and young people (younger than 25 years), and where possible, to meta-analyze data on the associations.

An electronic literature search was conducted for all studies published between January 1, 1996, and February 3, 2017, across sources, including MEDLINE, Cochrane, and PsycINFO. Articles of good quality were included if the study examined any association between cyber bullying involvement and self-harm or suicidal behaviors and reported empirical data in a sample aged under 25 years. A total of 33 eligible articles from 26 independent studies were included, covering a population of 156,384 children and young people. A total of 25 articles (20 independent studies, n=115,056) identified associations (negative influences) between cyber victimization and self-harm or suicidal behaviors or between perpetrating cyber bullying and suicidal behaviors. Three additional studies, in which the cyber bullying, self-harm, or suicidal behaviors measures had been combined with other measures (such as traditional bullying and mental health problems), also showed negative influences (n=44,526). A total of 5 studies showed no significant associations (n=5646). Meta-analyses, producing odds ratios (ORs) as a summary measure of effect size (e.g, ratio of the odds of cyber victims who have experienced non victims who have experienced SH), showed that, compared with non-victims, those who have experienced cyber victimization were OR 2.35 (95% CI 1.65-3.34) times as likely to self-harm, OR 2.10 (95% CI 1.73-2.55) times as likely to exhibit suicidal behaviors, OR 2.57 (95% CI 1.69-3.90) times more likely to attempt suicide, and OR 2.15 (95% CI 1.70-2.71) times more likely to have suicidal thoughts. Cyber bullying perpetrators were OR 1.21 (95% CI 1.02-1.44) times more likely to exhibit suicidal behaviors and OR 1.23 (95% CI 1.10-1.37) times more likely to experience suicidal ideation than non-perpetrators.

The conclusion was that victims of cyber bullying are at a greater risk than non victims of both self-harm and suicidal behaviors.

Key findings from the Center's surveys of 743 teens and 1,058 parents living in the U.S. conducted March 7 to April 10, 2018 indicate throughout the report, that "teens" of ages 13 to 17 "of boys and girls have been harassed online but girls are more likely to be the targets of online rumor-spreading or nonconsensual explicit messages. The vast majority of teens (90% in this case) believe online harassment is a problem that affects people their age, and 63% say this is a major problem (Anderson, 2018).

Victims of cyberbullying have lower self-esteem, higher levels of depression, behavioral problems, substance abuse and experience significant life challenges (Hamm 2015 & Tokunanga, 2010). Ferrara et al (2014) observe that bullying victimization may trigger a sequence of events that results in suicidal behavior; Ferrara et al. identified in Italy 55 cases of suicide among children and young adults <18-year-old between January 2011 and December 2013 and 4 (7.3%) were bullying victims. After several suicides were linked to cyber bullying, media attention to such cases gradually increased, becoming more intense in recent years Aboujaoude et al (2015).

3.   Materials and Methods

3.1. Purpose of the Study

The purpose of the study was to establish risk factors and prevalence of suicidal behaviour among Kenyan youth due to worrying trend frequently reported suicide cases amongst young people in Kenya.

3.2 Objectives and Hypotheses of the Study

The study was guided by the objective that intended to examine the relationship between suicidal behaviour, family incidences, academic stress and depression among secondary school students .Based on the review of related literature, the following hypotheses were postulated and tested.

The Null (Ho) hypothesis: There is statistically insignificantly relationship between risk factors (family incidences, academic stress and depression) with suicidal behaviour among secondary school students in Busia County.

The Alternative (Ha) hypothesis: There is statistically significantly relationship between risk factors (family incidences, academic stress and depression) with suicidal behaviour among secondary school students in Busia County.

3.3 Study Population

We collected data from secondary school students in Busia County. Busia county has been hit by a wave youth suicidal attempts. It is located in western Kenya bordering Eastern Uganda. Students in this county come from all over the country since being a border county people from other parts of Kenya have settled in the area attract by cross- border economy.

3.4 Sample Size and Sampling Technique

To obtain a representation of schools in Busia County we first put schools into three clusters. One school was then selected from each cluster selected. For each school selected, stratified random sampling via gender, class and age were used was used to select the participants. Then, we estimated the sample size based on the number of students in each of the three

13

schools and choose 200 students. The samples were stratified into form one, form, two from three and form four students. The sampled schools were all mixed boys and girls. All students in the selected classes were invited to participate in the study. This study adopted a cross-sectional survey research design that made use of four scales to collect quantitative data from the participants.

3.5 Measures

Suicidal behavior in the future. The responses can be used to identify at risk individuals and specific risk behaviours. Item 1 is scored on 6-Likert scale; Item 2 on 5-Likert scale; Item 3 on 4 Likert scale and Item 4 on 7-Likert scale. Higher score is indicative of high ideation thoughts and behavior.

3.6 Consent for Participants

Permission for conducting research and data was sought and obtained for the researchers prior to data collection in schools. Written parental consent was sought since participants were under the age for self-consent in Kenya. However, researchers explained to the students the purpose of the study regarding their participation, as well as assure the students' responses were kept anonymous and confidential. Participation was strictly voluntary and students' responses were kept anonymous as they were instructed not to write their names.

3.7 Data Analysis

Data collated were analyzed using hierarchical multiple regressions analysis with the aid of statistical package for social sciences (SPSS: version 20). Descriptive statistics were used to determine the quantity and percentage distributions. To obtain the influence of suicidal risk factors on suicidal behaviour we first used a factor analysis and then included the significant factors in a multivariate logistic regression. Throughout the process, the p value was set at 0.05, and 95% confidence intervals were calculated.

4. Results and Discussions

In the bivariate analysis Table 1 presents the correlation matrix of all variables in the present study.

Table 1: Correlation matrix of suicide behaviour and risk factors

		SB	FD	DP	AS
	Pearson correlation		-.095	.321**	.092
Suicide behaviour (SB)	Sig (s-tailed		.186	.000	.201
	N		196	196	196
	Pearson correlation	-.095		-.220**	.013
Family Dysfunctions (FD)	Sig (s-tailed	.186		.002	.854
	N	196		196	196
	Pearson correlation	.321**	-.220**		.315**
Depression (DP)	Sig (s-tailed	.000	.002		.000
	N	196	196		196
	Pearson correlation	.092	.013	.315**	
Academic stress (AS)	Sig (s-tailed	.201	.854	.000	
	N	196	196	196	

** Correlation is significant at the 0.01 level (2-tailed)

A Pearson product- moment correlation coefficient was conducted to examine the relationships between suicidal behaviour, family dysfunctions, academic stress and depression among secondary school students. Suicidal behaviour was moderately positively correlated to depression, r (196) = .321, P < 0.01, than to family values, r(196)= -.095, P > 0.01 and academic stress, r(196) = .092, P> 0.01. These findings suggest that depression explained much more of the variability in suicidal behaviour than does family dysfunctions and academic stress. The effect size of depression (r^2 =.102) indicated that the level of depression the students experienced accounted for a small proportion (10.2%) variability in suicidal behaviour.

Adolescent depression was both positively correlated with family variables (r = 0.222, P < 0.01, and academic stress (r = 0.315, P < 0.01 with effect size of (r2 =.0492) for family values

15

and (r2 =.099) for academic stress. This implies the level of family values and academic stress that students experienced accounted for a small proportion of variance of 4.9% and 9.9% respectively.

4. Discussions

The objective of this study was to examine the relationship between suicidal behaviour, family incidences, academic stress and depression among secondary school students.

4:1 Suicidal behavior and families

In this study results suggested that suicidal behaviour is not influenced with family variable and academic stress. This further implies that youth may experience positive or negative responses from family but may not lead them towards suicidal thought. Although family variable and academic stress insignificantly influenced suicidal behaviour, focusing exclusively on depression in intervention programme may have limited effectiveness especially in African societies where youths with suicidal behaviour due to family dysfunctions and academic stress are less likely to reveal this to others as compared to their counterparts in the western world.

Forte (2018), in their research found the reverse in a few cases. The risk factors were found to be: family separation, language barriers, worrying about family back home and separation from family, often leading to hopelessness, depression, and anxiety. Furthermore, the lack of information on the health care system, loss of status, loss of social network, as well as acculturation when an individual acquires attitudes, etc. from a different country were identified as potential triggers to suicide. In china, factors identified with suicidal ideation include poor family structure and parental relationship (SAMHSA, 2012).

Macharia (2013) observed that adolescents also learned suicidal behaviour from family members. Mental health experts, assert that increased rate of attempted suicide cases among young people in Kenya is due to limited   capacity to think, act and process emotion in a rational manner especially when exposed to unbearable pressure, stress, drugs and alcohol.

Magaya et al (2005), in a study among a sample of Zimbabwean adolescents, found out that cultural factors bear a significant influence on adolescents' choice of coping approaches, as adolescents are often encouraged to adopt non-confrontational and avoidant behaviors that are focused on the promotion of a harmonious and interdependent social environment. This may

16

result into bottling up anger, unvented rage and suicidal ideation. Though this study was done in Zimbabwe, the Kenyan communities, especially in the rural areas bring up their children in a similar way. It would therefore be important to find out whether teachers know that how students have been socialized to deal with stressing events is related to suicidal behavior.

4.2 Suicidal behavior and academics

Academic stress may also not directly lead to suicidal behaviour. This is similar to Kerr et al (2011) who revealed that family issues and academic stress insignificantly accounted for the suicidal ideation in adolescents. Suicidal behaviour was negatively correlated with family variable and academic stress. This concurred with Aboujaoude et al (2015), who stated that cyber bullying should also be considered as a cause for new onset psychological symptoms, somatic symptoms of unclear etiology or a drop in academic performance. In addition, Macharia (2013) in a study on suicidal behavior risk factors of secondary schools adolescents in Nyandarua, Kenya, found that parent-child communication, dysfunctional families, irresponsible parenting, absence of parents and parents pressure on adolescents to perform academically were risk factors that fuelled suicide ideation among adolescents.

Symptoms readily observed in the school setting that may affect academics include an inability to concentrate, to think rationally, or make even minor decisions; other observable symptoms include difficulty getting necessary things done, self-harm behavior, withdrawing from normal relationships or isolating oneself, and increased absenteeism in school (Klein et al., 2013). Such problems may be reflected in students' classroom behavior, homework habits, and academic performance (Hubert, 2006).

4.3 Suicidal behavior and depression

Adolescent depression significantly influenced suicidal behaviour. The results suggested that depressed mood increases with suicidal behaviour for youth in this sample. This is similar to Kerr et al (2011) in their findings indicated that depression significantly accounted for the suicidal ideation in youth. In another study victims of cyber bullying were found to have lower self-esteem, higher levels of depression, behavioral problems, substance abuse and experience significant life challenges which may lead to suicidal thoughts (Hamm 2015;

Tokunanga, 2010). The conclusion was that victims of cyberbullying are at a greater risk than non victims of both self-harm and suicidal behaviors.

In another study done in Kenya it was observed that suicidal behaviour is a common problem among youths identified with psychiatric or substance abuse disorder (Lincoln et al, 2013). Cleare et al, (2018) state that adverse childhood experiences have been implicated in a range of negative health outcomes in adulthood, including mental disorders and suicide death. It was observed that adolescents who struggle with suicidal behavior often exhibit unhealthy thought patterns due to mental health issues such as depression, that lead to thoughts of hopelessness, helplessness, and worthlessness (SAMHSA, 2012). Handley et al, (2018) found out from the Australian Rural Mental Health Study that, of 1051 participants, 364 reported life-time depression leading to suicide. This revealed a relationship between depression and suicidal behavior. In addition, certain risk factors depression, anxiety, and mental illness are common in all cultural groups, as observed by Molock (2020), but these factors may present and be conceptualized differently across different cultures. Mental health and suicide prevention services must therefore be tailored creatively to the needs of each culture.

5.   Conclusions

The influence of family variables academic stress and depression on suicidal behaviour was examined in a sample of secondary school youths from Busia County. Family variables and, depression, questionnaires, academic stress and Suicidal Behavior Questionnaire Revised Scale were employed.   The depression questionnaire administered yielded statistically significant results while family variables and academic stress were statistically insignificant to youth suicidal behaviour, providing evidence in this sample that depression was of significant influence to youth suicidal behaviour. The present findings may imply intervention and prevention programmes with youth in schools to address issues of youth depressions.

Limitations of self-administered questionnaire, sole respondent and omitted variables were noted. Despite some of the shortcomings, this study has extended research by specifically testing the association of family variables, academic stress, depression and suicidal behaviour among the youth. This general methodological approach may be generalized to other areas of study within youth mental health child and psychology.

6.   Recommendations

Need to offer suicide prevention education in schools and entire public to create awareness and optimal suicide prevention programmes in school and community. Part of the programme should be to initiate peer gatekeeper programs related to identifying at-risk peers and encouraging them to seek help from the counselors or therapeutic service providers.

Engage with support groups, family, friends, and other community members. Participate in community activities to prevent suicide thoughts and encourage strong connections to family, friends, and community support

Parents and teacher should prioritize interacting with youth in positive ways. Increase youth involvement in positive experiences and communications (i.e., texting, Facebook, Twitter) with the goal of keeping them safe

Policies on convicting cyber bullies be enacted to protect youth

Engage youth in skills of problem solving, conflict resolution and handling problems in a non-violent way.

7.   Limitations

There are a few limitations of the present study that should be noted. First, our data were based exclusively on students' self-administered questionnaire. It is possible that because youths were the sole respondents, insignificant associations obtained between family variables, academic stress and suicidal behaviour may reflect problems associated with shared opinion and intention to faking bad. Shared opinion may result in spuriously high correlations among constructs. Future research could consider a multiple informant and multiple method strategy to overcome the problem of shared opinion.

The Second limitation of the current study is the focus on family variables academic stress and depression as independent variables of the relations with youth suicidal behaviour. It is possible that other variables not included in the present study could be of stronger influence to youth suicidal. Also, the strong association between the depression and suicidal behaviour may be due other variables not covered in the study.

8. References

Aboujaoude E, Savage MW, Starcevic V, Salame WO. Cyberbullying: review of an old problem gone viral. J Adolesc Health. 2015 Jul;57(1):10–8

Anderson, M. (2018) Cyber bulling Https://www.pewresearch.org/staff monica-anderson *Annual   Review of Clinical Psychology* 2, 237-266. retrieved on 17 April 2020 03.45am

Ann John1, FFPH ; Alexander Charles Glendenning1, ; Amanda Marchant1, ; Paul Montgomery, DPhil ; Anne Stewart, FRCPsych ; Sophie Wood1,; Keith Lloyd1, FRCPsych ; Keith Hawton, FMedSci Self-Harm, Suicidal Behaviours, and Cyberbullying in Children and Young People: Systematic Review https://www.jmir.org/search/searchResultfield=author&criteria 15April 03.00am

Bachmann S. Epidemiology of Suicide and the Psychiatric Perspective. Int. J. Environ. Res. Public Health. 2018;15:1425. doi: 10.3390/ijerph15071425. [PMC free article] [PubMed] [CrossRef] [Google Scholar]

Bullismo in Italia: comportamenti Offensivie violent tra I giovanissimi http:// www./stat.it/it/files/2015/12/bullismo.pdf?title=bullismo ++tra accessed 28 nov 2017

Brådvik,L. (2018). Suicide Risk and Mental Disorders http://www.nbci.nim.nih.gov/pmc/articles PMC 6165520/# B 1-ijerph - 15- 02028

Cash, S.J. & Bridge, J.A. (2009) Epidemiology of youth suicide and suicidal behavior. *Current*

Cavanagh J.T., Carson A.J., Sharpe M., Lawrie S.M. Psychological autopsy studies of suicide: A systematic review. Psychol. Med. 2003;33:395–405. do10.1017/S0033291702006943. [PubMed] [CrossRef] [Google Scholar]

Cleare S., Wetherall K., Clark A., Ryan C., Kirtley O.J., Smith M., O'Connor R.C. Adverse Childhood Experiences and Hospital-Treated Self-Harm. Int. J. Environ. Res. Public Health. 2018;15:1235. doi: 10.3390/ijerph15061235. [PMC free article] [PubMed] [CrossRef] [Google Scholar]

Commissariato di PS, Una Vita da social Https:// www.commissariatodips. It/upload/media/ communicato_Stampa_una_vita_da_social_4_edizione_2017. Accessed 28 Nov 2019

Crona L., Stenmarker M., Öjehagen A., Asklund U., Brådvik L. Taking care of oneself by regaining control—A key to staying alive four to five decades after a suicide attempt in severe depression. BMC

Crona L., Stenmarker M., Öjehagen A., Asklund U., Brådvik L.(2017). Taking care of oneself by regaining control—A key to staying alive four to five decades after a suicide attempt in severe depression. BMC Psychiatry. 2017;17:69. doi: 10.1186/s12888-017-1223-4. [PMC free article] [PubMed] [CrossRef] [Google Scholar]

Culbreth, R., Swahn, M.H., Ndetei, D., Ametewee, L.,& Kasirye, R. (2018). Suicidal Ideation among Youth Living in the Slums of Kampala, Uganda International journal of environmental research and public health

Eaton, D.K., Kann, L., Kinchen, S., Shanklin, S., Ross, J., Hawkins, J., Harris, W.A., Lowry, R.,

Ferrara P., Lanniello F.,Cutrona C., Quintarelli F., Vena F. Del Volgo V. et al. (2014). A Focus on recent cases of suicides among Italian children & adolescent and a review of literature. Ital J. Pediatr 2014 July 15: 40:69

Forte A., Trobia F., Gualtieri F., Lamis D.A., Cardamone G., Giallonardo V., Fiorillo A., Girardi P., Pompili M.(2018). Suicide Risk among Immigrants and Ethnic Minorities: A Literature Overview. Int. J. Environ. Res. Public Health. 2018;15:1438.doi: 10.3390/ijerph15071438. [PMC free article] [PubMed] [CrossRef] [Google Scholar

Hamm M.P. Newton A.S., Chisholm A., Shulhan J. Milne A. Sundar P. et al (2015). Prevalence & effect of cyber bulling on children and young people a scoping review of social media studies. JAMA pediatr, 2015 Aug 169(8): 770-7

Handley T., Rich J., Davies K., Lewin T., Kelly B. (2018). The Challenges of Predicting Suicidal Thoughts and Behaviours in a Sample of Rural Australians with Depression. Int. J. Environ. Res. Public Health. 2018;15:928. doi: 10.3390/ijerph15050928. [PMC free article] [PubMed] [CrossRef] [Google Scholar]

Hawton K., Casañas I., Comabella C., Haw C., Saunders K.(2013). Risk factors for suicide in individuals with depression: A systematic review. J. Affect. Disord. 2013;147:17–28. doi: 10.1016/j.jad.2013.01.004. [PubMed] [CrossRef] [Google Scholar]

Heu U., Bogren M., Wang A.G., Brådvik L. (2018).Son between Suicides and Controls and General Pattern. Int. J. Environ. Res. Public Health. 2018;15:1299. doi: 10.3390/ijerph15071299. [PMC free article] [PubMed] [CrossRef] [Google Scholar]

Holmstrand C., Bogren M., Mattisson C., Brådvik L. (2015). Long-term suicide risk in people with no, one or more mental disorders: The Lundby study 1947–1997. Acta Psychiatr. Scand. 2015;132:459–469. doi: 10.1111/acps.12506. [PMC free article] [PubMed] [CrossRef] [Google Scholar]

Huberty, T. (2006). *Depression: Helping students in the classroom*. Retrieved fromhttp://www.nasponline.org/publications/cq/index-list.aspx.1080/13811110802101203

Hui Zhai & Bing Bai (2015). Correlation between Family Environment and Suicidal Ideation in University Students in China. *International Journal of Environmental Research and Public Health, (12),* 1412-1424

Iemmi V., Bantjes J., Coast E., Channer K., Leone T., McDaid D., Palfreyman A., Stephens B., Lund C.(2016)/ Suicide and poverty in low-income and middle-income countries: A systematic review. Lancet Psychiatry. 2016;3:774–783. doi: 10.1016/S2215-0366(16)30066-9. [PubMed] [CrossRef] [Google Scholar]

Inskip H., Harris E.C., Barraclough B.(1998). Lifetime risk of suicide for affective disorder, alcoholism and schizophrenia. Br. J. Psychiatry. 1998; 172:35–37. doi: 10.1192/bjp.172.1.35. [PubMed] [CrossRef] [Google Scholar]

Kerr M., Engels R.C.M., Overbreek G. Andershed A-K, Stattin (2011). Understanding Girls Problem Behaviour: How girls Deliquency develops in the context of maturity & health; co-occuring problems & relationships. Edited .John Willey & Sons Ltd . USA

Khasakhala, L. L., Ndetei, D. M., & Mathai, M. (2013). Suicidal behavior among youths associated with psychopathology in both parents and youths attending outpatient psychiatric clinic in Kenya. *Annals of General Psychiatry, 12*(13), 1-8

Khasakhala, L., Sorsdahl, K. R., Harder, V. S., Williams, D. R., & Ndetei, D. M. (2011). Lifetime mental disorders and suicidal behavior in South Africa. *African Journal of Psychiatry*

King C.A., Merchant C.R. (2008). Social and Interpersonal Factors Relating to Adolescent Suicidality: A Review of the Literature. Arch. Suicide Res. 2008;12:181–196. doi: 10 [PMC free article] [PubMed] [CrossRef] [Google Scholar]

Klein, D.N., Kujawa, A.J., Black, S.R., & Pennock, A.T. (2013). Depressive disorders. In Beauchaine, T.P. & Hinshaw, S.P. (Eds.), *Child and Adolescent Psychopathology* (2nd ed.) (pp. 543-575). Hoboken, NJ: John Wiley & Sons

Lincoln I., Khasakhala, L.I., Ndetei, D.M. & Muthoni, M. (2013). *Suicidal behaviour among youths associated with psychopathology in both parents and youths attending outpatient psychiatric clinic in Kenya.* Annals of General Psychiatry 2013, 12:13 http://www.annals-general-psychiatry.com/content/12/1/13

Linehan, M. M. (2015). *DBT skills training manual.* New York: The Guilford Press.

Macharia, A. M. (2013). *Teachers' Knowledge of Identify Suicidal Behavior Risk Factors of Adolescents in Public Secondary Schools in Nyandarua South District, Nyandarua County, Kenya* (Master's Thesis). Catholic University of Eastern Africa, Kenya

Magaya, L. Asner-Self, K. K., & Schreiber, J. B. (2005). Stress and coping among Zimbabwean adolescents. *British Journal of Educational Psychology, 22,* 36-47

McManus, T., Chyen, D., Lim, C., Brener, N.D. & Wechsler, H. (2008) Youth risk behavior surveillance--United States, 2007. *MMWR Surveillance Summaries* 57, 1-131.

Mérelle S., Foppen E., Gilissen R., Mokkenstorm J., Cluitmans R., Van Ballegooijen W. (2018). Characteristics Associated with Non-Disclosure of Suicidal Ideation in Adults. Int. J. Environ. Res. Public Health. 2018;15:943. doi: 10.3390/ijerph15050943. [PMC free article] [PubMed] [CrossRef] [Google Scholar]

Miller, A. L., Rathus, J. H., & Linehan, M. M. (2007). Dialectical behavior therapy with suicidal adolescents. Guilford Press.

Mokkenstorm J., Franx G., Gilissen R., Kerkhof A., Smit J.H. (2018). Suicide Prevention Guideline Implementation in Specialist Mental Healthcare Institutions in The Netherlands. Int. J. Environ. Res. Public Health. 2018;15:910. doi: 10.3390/ijerph15050910. [PMC free article] [PubMed] [CrossRef] [Google Scholar]

Molock, et al (2020). On Mental Health and Culture Suicide Among Adolescents. https://www.psychiatryadvisor.com/home/topic/suicide-and-self-harm/ 2020;03:42am

Ndetei, D. M., Pizzo, M., Khasakhala, L. L., Mutiso, V. N., Ongecha, F. A., & Kokonya, D. Ndetei, K., Mutiso A.V., Mbwayo, A. M and Mathai, M. (2011). The prevalence of depression among adolescents in Nairobi public secondary schools: association with perceived maladaptive parenting behavior. *African Journal of Psychiatry.* Department of Psychiatry, University of Nairobi, Nairobi, Kenya

Ng L.C., Kirk C.M., Kanyanganzi F., Fawzi M.C.S., Sezibera V., Shema E., Bizimana J.I., Cyamatare F.R., Betancourt T.S.(2015). Risk and protective factors for suicidal ideation and behaviour in Rwandan children. Br. J. Psychiatry J. Ment. Sci. 2015;207:262–268. doi: 10.1192/bjp.bp.114.154591. [PMC free article] [PubMed] [CrossRef] [Google Scholar

Omigbodun, O., Dogra, N., Esan, O., & Adedokun, B. (2008). Prevalence and correlates of suicidal behavior among adolescents in Southwest Nigeria. *International Journal of Social Psychiatry, 54*(1), 34-46.*Opinion in Pediatrics* 21, 613-619.

Page R.M., West J.H. (2011). Suicide Ideation and Psychosocial Distress in Sub-Saharan African Youth. Am. J. Health Behav. 2011;35:129–141. doi: 10.5993/AJHB.35.2.1. [PubMed] [CrossRef] [Google Scholar]

Palmier, J. B. (2011). *Prevalence and correlates of suicidal ideation among students in sub-Saharan African* (Unpuplished master's thesis*).* Atlantis: USA: Georgia State University

Magaya, Asner-Self and Schreiber (2005). Prevalence and correlates of suicidal ideation and physical fighting: A comparison of students in Botswana, Kenya, Uganda, Zambia and United States. *International Public Health Journal, 172*(24), 151-162.*Psychiatry, 14*(2), 134-139 NO

Schlebusch, L., Burrows, S. & Vawda, N. (2009). *Suicide prevention and religious traditions on the African continent.* Oxford England: Oxford University Press

Spirito, A. & Esposito-Smythers, C. (2006) Attempted and completed suicide in adolescence. Substance Abuse and Mental Health Services Administration (SAMHSA). (2012). *Preventing suicide: A toolkit for high schools.* HHS Publication No. SMA-12- 4669. Rockville, MD: Center for Mental Health Services, Substance Abuse and Mental Health Services Administration

Swahn M.H., Palmier J.B., Kasirye R., Yao H. (2012). Correlates of Suicide Ideation and Attempt among Youth Living in the Slums of Kampala. Int. J. Environ. Res. Public Health. 2012;9:596–609. doi: 10.3390/ijerph9020596. [PMC free article] [PubMed] [CrossRef] [Google Scholar]

Tanney, B. L. (1992). Mental disorders, psychiatric patients, and suicide. In R. W. Maris, A. L. Berman, J. T. Maltsberger, & R. I. Yufit (Eds.), *Assessment and prediction of suicide* (p. 277–320). Guilford Press

Tokunanga (2020), Following your home from school: A critical review and synthesis of research on cyber bullying victimization. Comput Hum Behav, 2010: 26: 277- 87

Tom, F. , Kate, G.& Roy,M. (2028). Mental disorders and suicide in Northern
Ireland. https://doi.org/10.1192/bjp.170.5.447 Published online by Cambridge
University Press: 03 January 2018

World Health Organization [WHO]. (2019). *World Suicide Prevention Day "Working
Together To Prevent Suicide" to highlight the most essential ingredient for effective
global suicide prevention. 10 September 2019. International Association for Suicide
Prevention*www.unicef.org/publications

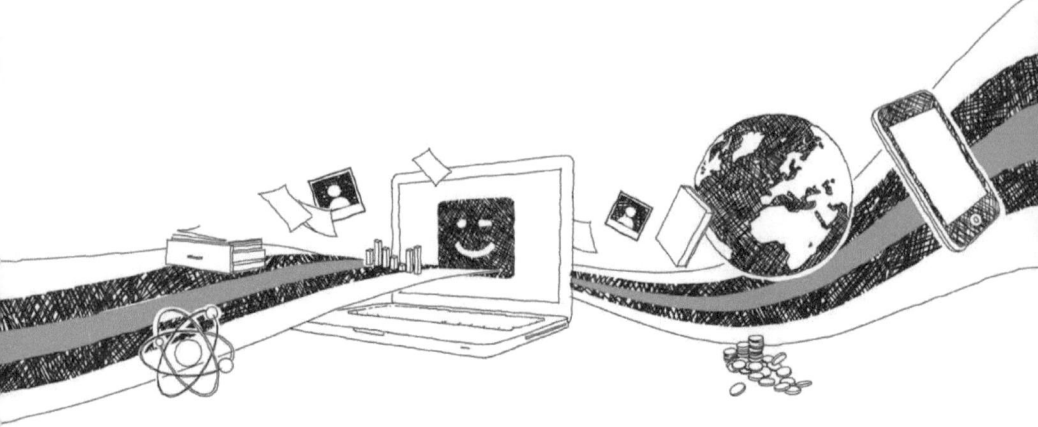
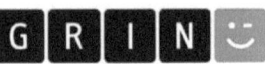